THE **RESIDENCY INTERVIEW**

How To Make the Best Possible Impression

Jessica Freedman, MD

ISBN: 0615325920

ISBN-13: 9780615325927

Library of Congress Control Number: 2010922471

AUTHOR'S NOTE:

Some of the anecdotes I have used in this book are based on my actual experiences but applicants' identities have been concealed. Some of this material, including the sample interview, is completely fictitious. Remember that plagiarism is illegal so do not regurgitate any of the information provided in this book for your actual interview or in your application materials. Authenticity is essential for your success so even if you aren't "caught," doing so will jeopardize your chances of matching. The information provided in this book does not guarantee that you will obtain a residency position.

CONTENTS

PART I
ANATOMY OF THE RESIDENCY INTERVIEW

PART 2
INTERVIEW PREPARATION AND FOLLOW UP

APPENDICES

ABOUT THE AUTHOR

Jessica Freedman, MD is a former associate residency director and faculty member at the Mount Sinai School of Medicine in New York City. A top rated faculty member at Mount Sinai, she was involved in medical education and curriculum design at the graduate and undergraduate levels. She is also a published author and has served on national committees related to medical education. Dr. Freedman is now president of MedEdits, a private advising company for applicants to medical school, residency and fellowship. Dr. Freedman is a practicing emergency physician and lives in New Jersey.

INTRODUCTION

I started my "interview career" as an interviewee myself when I was a premedical student and then again as a residency applicant, but I learned most about this process during the 10 years I spent in the interviewer's seat. I started interviewing residency applicants as a senior emergency medicine resident and continued throughout my tenure as a residency admissions officer. Like most physicians, I had no formal training or experience when I started interviewing candidates. During my years of selecting candidates, I learned what qualities applicants must have to interview well. More important, however, I learned what goes on behind the scenes after interview day and how a candidate's success is affected by the interviewer's skills and experience. Indeed, I gained an understanding of how both experienced and inexperienced interviewers evaluate applicants and what applicants can do to influence these differences to their advantage. After working with applicants who are preparing for interviews with www.MedEdits. com, I also know what common mistakes interviewees make. These experiences, from both the "outside" and the "inside," allow me to provide a unique perspective to medical students and medical school graduates who are preparing for interviews. Thus, this book, based on my inside understanding of the residency admissions process and my work privately advising clients, is a must-read for both interviewees and interviewers alike.* It covers everything you need to know, beginning with what you should do to prepare for interview day, what to expect on The Day, and the nitty gritty of how to behave during and after the interview. By having a full understanding of the residency admissions process, knowing what goes on behind the scenes before and after your interview, who will be interviewing you, what the interviewer is looking for and what you can do to influence how your interview will progress, you will be better prepared to do well and present yourself in the best light.

*A NOTE FOR THE INTERVIEWER

I encourage residency interviewers to read this book since you may gain some insight into how to interview residency candidates to make thorough, accurate and complete assessments. I find that many resident interviewers and first time attending interviewers are often as nervous as the applicants! Based on my own experience in academic medicine, I know that we typically receive no training on how to interview applicants. In fact, I sometimes found myself teaching my senior attendings about how to review an application and interview an applicant to make sure all important information was obtained and to rule out any red flags.

There are always applicants who have "slipped through the cracks" when the admissions committee failed to notice a significant piece of their history. These applicants may have difficulty in residency or as attendings, and it is therefore the interviewer's responsibility to make sure such individuals are identified. Failure to do so may compromise a seat in a program when a resident cannot complete a portion of his or her training and may also negatively impact patient care. I work primarily with candidates, but I have also helped friends and colleagues to refine and improve their interviewing and application reviewing skills.

CHAPTER 1: **THE INTERVIEW PROCESS**

Typically only one to three people per program are responsible for screening residency applications, and how they do it is important to understand. Since some programs may have up to 500 (or even 1,000) applications for only 100 interview slots, for example, it becomes the responsibility of those reviewing applications to decide who will be invited. I can tell you from experience that making these decisions is a daunting task. To decrease the work load, many program directors apply filters to applications to decrease the number of applications that must be reviewed to a reasonable quantity. What kinds of "filters" are used? There are many. Some filters may be applied so program directors only review applications who have a certain United States Medical Licensing Exam (USMLE) step 1 score as a threshold, others may use a filter that only views applicants who have graduated within five years, while others may use no filters and manually review every application submitted. Some programs then assign "points" for everything: research, USMLE scores, and letters of recommendation; you are invited for an interview only when your "score" meets a minimum number. More often, however, a great deal of subjectivity goes into the decision to invite an applicant for an interview, whatever the grading system. Often, the screener's personal interests and outlook play a part in the review of your application--especially if you are a "borderline" applicant. For example, if reviewer A always had to struggle with standardized tests yet managed to succeed while reviewer B always had board scores in the top 5th percentile, reviewer A is much more likely than reviewer B to screen in an application with lower-than-average board scores.

The person reading your application might have years of admissions experience or he or she could be a novice, such as a junior faculty member or a very fresh assistant program director. Both the level of experience of the screener and his or her own biases and preferences often determine whether or not you are granted an interview. This is why norms for a program can change dramatically from year to year. If a new program director who is a Caribbean medical school graduate comes on board, for example, a program may suddenly become "Caribbean medical school graduate friendly" and may go from matching with no Caribbean medical students to filling 70% of their slots with them. Also, although the person reading your application might have hours to peruse through all of your materials, it is more likely that she is tired and rushed and has a large volume of applications to review. If your application follows one that is more stellar, yours may pale in comparison. On the other hand, if the pile contains mostly mediocre-to-poor applications, yours may stand out.

Most reviewers also review applications in a systematic way and everyone has their own style. Since applications are typically reviewed on a computer rather than a printed hard copy of your application, the reviewer can choose which portions of your application to review and in what order. When I reviewed applications as the associate program director, my preferred order was as follows:

1. Applicant's demographic information, including where he or she went to school.

2. USMLE scores. Even though I knew that these scores did not always predict who would be a good resident and I often felt guilty for considering them in my evaluation, it was the only way for me to compare "apples to apples" so it became an important factor.

3. Letters of reference, looking first at those from people whom I knew and from people within the specialty. I would then consider other letters of reference.

4. Grades.

5. Applicant's activities.

6. Personal statement.

7. Medical School Performance Evaluation (MSPE).

Based on my overall assessment, I would then decide if the applicant should be invited for an interview. But, if my decision was made after step 4 and I felt I had enough information to make a decision, I might only skim the applicant's other materials. For the applicant who was "on the fence," the activities descriptions, personal statement and MSPE became more important.

What is most important varies from reviewer to reviewer, however. But keep in mind that the 2008 Program Director Survey by the National Residency Matching Program indicates that the MSPE, grades, letters of reference, USMLE Step I/COMLEX score and personal statement are the top factors across all specialties.

Given all the applications administrators must review, making your application as distinctive as possible will increase the likelihood that you will be invited for an interview. If the application bores the person reviewing your application, he or she will likely click the "hold" or "rejection" box on the application system. But you must also understand that many applicants to residency are highly qualified and that many steps in the selection process are out of your control. This is a hard truth to accept, and you can only hope that your application and letters of reference are appealing enough to trigger some interview invitations. Each interview is a chance to be ranked highly, so it is essential to be prepared and know what to expect.

CHAPTER 2: **WHAT ARE THE DIFFERENT TYPES OF INTERVIEWS?**

You may not always know what type of interview is conducted for the program at which you are interviewing, and the type may vary from year to year depending on program leadership changes and from interviewer to interviewer. Below are the six major types of interviews.

Open file

An open file interview is the most common type of interview. In an open file interview, the interviewer has access to all of your information, including all written documents, letters of reference and test scores. But just because an interview is open file does not mean that the interviewer has read all of your materials. Your interview is just one part of his day, and if the interviewer was caring for patients before he sat down, he probably has not had time to read through your file. Or, maybe your interviewer was teaching a class that ran late, and he had only five minutes to review your materials. You must prepare for an open file interview in the same way you would for a closed file interview (discussed below). Do not assume that your interviewer knows a thing about you. Also, do not be offended if your interviewer reads your file while you are speaking. This may be the first time he has glimpsed at your personal statement, application and letters of reference.

Closed file interview or partial file interview

In this type of interview, the interviewer may have no or limited access to your materials. These interviews therefore offer an opportunity to control the interview and dictate what is discussed. In a closed file interview, the interviewer typically has access to your curriculum vitae and nothing else.

In practical terms, the vast majority of residency interviews should be considered closed file. Since most programs interview large numbers of applicants, many interviewers do not have time to review applications in advance.

Panel interview

Applicants tend to find a panel interview more intimidating than any other type. Typically, the panel comprises three interviewers and one interviewee. Or, there may be stations, each with its own panel of two or three interviewers. I had one interview like this during my own residency interview experience and, indeed, I found it very stressful. How this interview proceeds depends in part on the dynamic and hierarchy of the interviewers. For example, a junior faculty member may be intimidated by a more senior faculty member and therefore may be more concerned with her own performance than with the interviewee's. It is important during these interviews not to psychoanalyze the group who is interviewing you but to stay focused on their questions and your own personal agenda of what you hope to convey.

Group interview

These interviews typically involve several interviewers and interviewees. Their objective is to see how you manage pressure and how you respond to others. You should listen attentively to everyone's answers and be a team player. If someone gives an answer that you wanted to give, make a joke: "John just gave my answer and now I have nothing to say." Do not act as though the other interviewees are competitors. Listen respectfully to what they have to say, make eye contact and be interested in everyone. Though it is natural to compare yourself with other interviewees in the group, be aware that the other interviewees' answers may "sound better" than your own, not because they actually are superior to your answers, but because their stories are new to you.

Phone interviews

I find that these types of interviews are reserved for international medical graduates and mostly serve the purpose of screening applicants. The interviewer is trying to assess your communication skills. These interviews typically precede in-person interviews.

The skills interview

This interview type is rare and is typically reserved for the surgical specialties. Some programs have been known to ask applicants to perform a task, such as suturing, while being interviewed. The word "gets out" on these programs so you will likely have advance warning for this type of interview.

CHAPTER 3: **WHAT IS THE RESIDENCY INTERVIEWER LOOKING FOR?**

It is important to understand what interviewers are looking for within the context of your experience. Residency applicants often fail to make a good impression when they try to tell interviewers what they think they want to hear instead of representing themselves honestly and authentically. Since your grades, USMLE scores and letters of reference will be used to evaluate your academic aptitude, interviewers are trying to assess something else-- they want to know if you are really committed to the specialty to which you are applying, that you have a mature sense of what it means to practice your specialty and how good your interpersonal and communication skills are—among other attributes. Above all, interviewers are trying to assess your "fit" for a program. Residency is intense and you will be spending a lot of time with the individual interviewer, his colleagues and his residents. So, your interviewer is fundamentally trying to determine if he likes you and would be happy to see you at 3 AM when he is tired. Residency interviewers are not looking for the same subtleties that your medical school interviewers were; they assume that you want to be a doctor. You should, in part, view your residency interview as a job interview; they want to know that you can get the job done reliably and competently. Interviewers also want to rule out any red flags, such as gaps in time on your record, many changes in careers or interests or any signs of personal instability.

Do you have a demonstrated commitment to and understanding of the specialty to which you are applying?

Interviewers are trying to assess first and foremost your motivation to pursue your desired specialty. They want to hear about when and why you decided to pursue this specialty, and they want to know that your background justifies your claim that you want to practice this specialty. For example, if you are interviewing for a residency in anesthesiology, it won't be very convincing to the person interviewing you that you are committed if your only experience in anesthesiology was a two-week stint during your surgery rotation. In contrast, the person who has done that two-week stint plus two full rotations in the specialty and has more rotations planned later in the year that will prepare them for residency presents a much more convincing argument. Interviewers also want to know that you understand what you are getting yourself in to, that you understand the pros and cons of practicing your desired specialty and have a realistic idea of the challenges you will face. They will assess your understanding of what you will actually do in your desired specialty. Interviewers may also ask about health care reform and specifically how it may affect your specialty. They want to know that you aren't living in a cave and that you understand that reforms are likely in your future.

Do you have what it takes to make it through residency training and a future medical career?

It takes a tremendous amount of dedication, hard work, resilience and perseverance to do well in residency training, which can be very rigorous. With the exception of only a few specialties, residency demands functioning well despite working long hours and many nights and weekends. While interviewers will glean information about your strengths based on your letters of reference, they are also trying to assess these qualities during your interview. Residency training also presents intellectual, emotional and physical challenges that a medical student cannot appreciate. So, it is your interviewer's job to decide if you have the characteristics that make it likely you will be able to cope and succeed throughout your training and in your future career. They want to know that you will work hard, that you are emotionally stable and that you will be able to learn and apply what you will learn during your training.

Are you confident yet humble?

Even a hint of arrogance or self-righteousness might destroy your chances of being ranked. Humility is much preferred over self-centeredness and a fine line sometimes differentiates confidence from overconfidence. Be sure not to do anything that might suggest you are overconfident, for example, by acting too informal or familiar, appearing too comfortable, dropping names or obviously promoting yourself. Let your accomplishments speak for themselves and hope that your letter writers wrote about your positive qualities and attributes. An attending's greatest fear is to end up with a resident who is overconfident; such an individual may not be "teachable," which ultimately can jeopardize patient care.

Would the interviewers enjoy spending long periods of time with you?

In emergency medicine, we often asked ourselves, "Could I spend an 8 hour overnight shift with this person?" If the answer was "No way, he would really make me nuts," the applicant typically would not be ranked. The residency faculty will be your teachers, colleagues and even friends for three to five years. So, you must convince them that having you around would be comfortable and pleasant. This is why small talk matters during your interview day; interviewers want to know that you are personable and, bottom line, good company.

Can you recognize your faults and admit when you are wrong?

No one expects you to be perfect. In fact, program directors want to know that you can recognize your faults and that you can make improvements or modify your behaviors accordingly. Faculty members want to see that you have learned from any flaws they identify. They also want to know that you are aware of your limitations. An important part of being a great doctor is knowing when it is time to ask for help and to be aware of your own strengths, expertise and weaknesses. Having a resident who doesn't recognize her own limits can negatively impact patient care.

Is everything consistent?

Interviewers also want to make sure that what you have written in your application and how you present yourself "match." Misrepresentation in either your application or your interview makes a negative impression. Consistency in your story is key, and interviewers will try to identify themes in your background and during your interview.

Are you smart and intellectually curious?

You also are being evaluated on your intelligence, intellectual curiosity and your ability to think logically and critically. While you won't be asked medical questions at most interviews (see box: Concerns for the International Medical Graduate (IMG)), a skilled interviewer can assess your abilities based on how you reason through the questions that are asked.

What is your demeanor and how do you communicate?

Residency applicants are judged on whether they are articulate, poised, enthusiastic, mature and, bottom line, pleasant to be around. **The best applicants smile, make good eye contact and are engaging, interesting, enthusiastic and warm.** Be sure you aren't swayed by a negative interviewer. You should greet even the grouchy interviewer happily and warmly and don't allow them to "bring you down." People with "sparkling personalities" always do better on interviews than their more sullen, stone faced or negative peers. Since communication skills, great interpersonal skills and the ability to relate to people are necessary to practice any specialty, you may be dinged if your interviewer thinks you have difficulty in these areas. But, at the same time, you must be true to yourself because not doing so may hinder your success. If you are not a smiley, energetic, and enthusiastic person, trying to be this person on your interview will seem unnatural and will make you anxious, which will undermine your success. What is most important is that you communicate articulately and that you are personable.

What will you bring to the residency?

Some interviewers also evaluate how you will add to the learning environment of the residency program but, to some degree, this depends on the prestige of the program. While some programs are looking for "bodies" to take care of patients, the more prestigious programs want to be convinced that you will be an active participant during residency, whether that means taking on an educational or research project, participating in a departmental committee or trying to get involved on a national level.

Are you a good "fit" for the residency?

Program directors are seeking out applicants who are the best fit for their residency. For example, a smaller community-focused residency program may not be interested in the applicant with 10 original publications who wants to make research a part of her career. So, while one applicant may be the ideal resident for one program, she may not be the best fit for another. You therefore should study each program's website before you interview to have a sense of what it values and what kind of residents it is trying to attract. As already emphasized, who you are on interview day must match the person the program director reads (or will read) about in your application, but you can often spin your experiences a bit to conform to their ideal applicant. Programs also tend to have "personalities," especially if they are small, so interviewers will try to assess your fit for a program by consciously or subconsciously making this judgment. You can get a sense of a program's personality based on the program's presentation and tour and by the demeanor of the attendings and residents whom you meet.

Do you have any red flags?

The two most obvious red flags are gaps in time of longer than three months when you cannot account for your activities or frequent jumps in career without any real explanation for these changes. Both of these factors suggest a lack of commitment or some possible underlying problem. Applicants who cannot communicate or are extremely nervous or anxious also raise concern. Interviewers are also trying to identify any major personality disorder or psychopathology that may hinder a candidate's ability not only to interact with patients and colleagues but their ability to complete residency. Other common "red flags" include a low grade or USMLE score, or withdrawals from classes, but, typically, if you were invited for an interview, these issues were not considered major. That said, you should be able to give explanations for the flaws in your application without making excuses. Also, do not assume that everything in the past is "water under the bridge." If you gained acceptance to medical school yet had an undergraduate career where you jumped from school to school, for example, assume that someone will pick up on this. We have all been in situations where red flags have been missed by the admissions committees who preceded us, so a keen interviewer will not assume that your application has no underlying issues.

Have you overcome any significant hardship or adversity?

Students who have overcome significant obstacles, such as coming from an underserved area, having financial hardship or being the first in their family to go to college should be evaluated within this cohort of applicants. But residency programs are not as aware of the importance and significance of such challenges as medical schools are when they consider whom to admit. For this reason, be sure to bring up any obstacles you have overcome in success-fully pursuing a medical career. Box I summarizes the qualities and characteristics interviewers tend to evaluate.

Box I

WHAT QUALITIES AND CHARACTERISTICS DO INTERVIEWERS EVALUATE?

Commitment to your specialty
Understanding of your specialty
Motivation to pursue a career in your desired specialty
Enthusiasm for your specialty
Direct experience in your specialty
Experience in other disciplines related to your specialty
Work ethic
Reliability
Professionalism
Maturity
Interpersonal skills
Ability to communicate
Intellectual abilities
Intellectual curiosity
Scholarly pursuits
Level of compassion
Level of empathy
Warmth
Experience in research
Experience in teaching
Leadership ability
Ability to think critically and analytically
Ability to listen
Ability to answer difficult questions
Ability to work as a member of a team
Personality and overall disposition
Reactions to situations (Do you ever become impatient or react impulsively?)
Values
Ability to overcome obstacles and cope with adversity
Achievements that make you stand out
Level of initiative
Red flags

CHAPTER 4: **WHO WILL INTERVIEW YOU?**

Most interviews are conversational and biographical. You may be interviewed by faculty, residency leadership (including the program director and associate program director) and current residents. The number of interviews you have and the length of these interviews varies tremendously. Many of my clients this year, in specialties ranging from anesthesiology to psychiatry, report that they are having only two or three interviews per program and that each interview lasts only 10 minutes! But, more typically, interviews last 15 to 20 minutes, and you will be interviewed by two to four faculty/residents. Why are interviews becoming so short? Well, it takes a tremendous amount of time to interview candidates and program faculty have many responsibilities in addition to interviewing candidates. Nonetheless, it seems difficult to make a judgment about people in such a short period of time so it seems logical that ranking decisions for these programs must be made on other factors, such as USMLE scores and letters of reference and a person's "gut feeling" about an interviewee. However, the brevity of many interviews also points up the importance of having an understanding of what information you want to convey during your interview.

Because your interviewer is your advocate and the primary support for your candidacy, it is essential to get on her good side. She (or he) will "sell you" to the other faculty. Your interviewer typically makes or breaks your acceptance. If she thinks highly of you, you will be ranked highly, but if you don't make a good impression, she will not support you. Remember your interviewer is human and, most of the time, is not trying to "get you." She wants to find out about you as a person and if you will be a good fit for the program. Because you cannot predict or control who your interviewer will be, it is important to have broad appeal as an interviewee and prepare yourself for multiple scenarios.

Based on my experience working with many interviewers and many applicants, I find that the types of interviewers fall into eight general categories, each of which calls for a different candidate approach (see Box 2: Types of interviewers). But to direct an interview to your advantage, you need to try early in the interview not only to get a fix on which type of interviewer you have but her perspective and level of experience, which also will affect how your interview progresses. Because most residency interviewers receive no training in interviewing candidates they do not necessarily know how to evaluate you comprehensively and effectively, as do more experienced interviewers. Why is this important? Because these inexperienced interviewers (who are most likely to be certain of the types described in Box 2) tend to ask more questions and have a different approach than more seasoned interviewers.

Box 2

TYPES OF INTERVIEWERS

The Mentor

The mentor represents the typical medical educator. These interviewers tend to be relaxed yet serious and have a fair amount of experience interviewing candidates. These interviews tend to be relaxed, and you typically are asked basic questions about your background, interest in your specialty and motivations. These interviewers are confident in their abilities, are committed to graduate medical education and may have extensive experience working with medical students and residents. They understand that the best way to gain the greatest understanding of an applicant's motivations, intelligence and character is if the candidate is relaxed. Their questions therefore tend to be basic and predictable. In general, the interviews they conduct are "easy." Mentor type interviewers tend to be residency directors or former residency directors.

The Professor

These interviewers can, based on appearance, seem to be the most intimidating when, in reality, they are usually great interviewers. Chairpeople and heads of departments tend to fall in this category. They are very experienced, have worked in different settings, have interviewed many candidates, residents and attendings, and have a vast amount of experience. They know what they are looking for and how to get the information they need and are typically efficient in seeking it out. Thus, your interviewer with the professor may veer off in another direction; you may start talking in depth about your research or your interest in philosophy or medical anthropology. Unlike the question shooter and the inappropriate interviewer (see below), however, the professor typically goes off on a tangent because he has effectively and efficiently assessed your candidacy and therefore has time to spare. He is confident in his abilities and can therefore get off topic. In some ways, the professor is the interviewer you want; he typically has a strong political voice on the faculty and, therefore, if he supports your candidacy can be a tremendous advocate. But, the reverse is also true; if he is not in favor of you, his opinion will also weigh heavily.

The "Sure, I'll Do It" Type

The "sure, I'll do it" interviewer is the person who was asked by his chairperson to serve on the residency admissions committee or was pulled in at the last minute when an interviewer was desperately needed. You are most likely to have this type of interviewer if the program is large or disorganized. Such programs often send out last-minute urgent emails to entire faculties begging for interviewers. Obviously, the type of interviewer you end up with in this situation is anybody's guess. He is usually participating because he thinks he "should" or because he thinks interviewing may be fun—which could mean the interviewer will have a relaxed attitude. In any case, it is unlikely that this interviewer is fully invested in the process and thus may be fairly malleable. Or, he may be completely clueless and have no idea how to interview. These interviews tend to be fairly undirected. The issue with the "sure I'll do it" interviewer is that you must provide the interviewer with the information that you know is important. These interviewers tend to be the greatest pushovers of all of the interviewer types, but they also may not be the strongest advocates. Thus, it is important to arm them with information about you and your motivations that they otherwise might not ask about.

The 5 Minute Interviewer

As mentioned earlier in this book, I am finding that more and more applicants are having interviews that last only 5 to 10 minutes. During this brief encounter, your interviewer may ask you just one specific question, which you should listen to carefully and answer just as specifically. But sometimes the interviewer only wants to know what questions or concerns you may have about the program. This is why you must have a few questions on hand. Some suggestions are discussed elsewhere in this book. Typically, however, these brief encounters are with the program director, who wants to ensure that he meets every interviewee.

The Question Shooter

This is most applicants' worst nightmare. This interviewer might ask you what three people you would like to invite to dinner and why.

He may also ask you about your greatest strength and weakness or ask you a very unusual question. Typically, the question shooter is inexperienced and asks questions because, bottom line, he doesn't know how to interview. He thinks asking random questions is what he is supposed to do and isn't even sure of the answers he is hoping to hear or how to evaluate your response. In some ways, these are the toughest interviews because you can in no way rely on your interviewer to ask you about what you want to tell him. The best way to manage these interviewers is to try and guide the interview. Make segues. Bring up topics you hope to discuss that highlight your strengths. (How to guide your interview will be discussed again later on in this book.)

The Inappropriate Interviewer
You are unlikely to have this type of interviewer because she usually doesn't last for long on admissions committees. Typically, an applicant complains and this interviewer is asked to leave the committee. You can spot an eccentric interviewer by the way she asks you sensitive or even illegal questions, often boring into the most sensitive topic in your background and delving into it. These interviewers are insensitive and think that by "digging" they will gain more information about your character or motivations. They may also ask you illegal questions about your personal family goals. Again, the best way to cope with these interviewers is to try and guide your interview and bring up topics you would like to discuss. When asked a question that you think may be illegal, such as a question about your sexuality, family plans or religion, it is best to answer vaguely and to try and change the topic. If you are really offended by an interviewer's questions, you should tell the program director about your experience and request another interview.

The Egomaniac
Ah, the egomaniacs. They are tough nuts to crack. They are generally young (or may be residents) and inexperienced, and they are psyched to be in a position of power. They think they have your life in their hands, and they have told all of their friends that they are on the residency admissions committee. They proclaim to all that

they are important. In some ways, the egomaniac is the toughest interviewer to impress, and it is not unusual for the egomaniac to want to hear himself speak as much as he wants to hear you speak. You cannot rely on the egomaniac to ask you about factors that will be relevant to your candidacy so you must guide your interview, and be sure to impart the information that you know is important.

The Strong Silent Type
The strong silent type likes to listen. These interviewers also may not like to ask too many questions. These types are rare since, in general, those who are shy do not typically volunteer to be on admissions committees. These interviewers are most challenging for shy applicants, and I envision a very quick interview when they get together. Your major concern if you get a strong silent type is that he is unlikely to loudly advocate for you during a residency admissions committee meeting.

CHAPTER 5: **MAKING THE MOST OF THE INTERVIEW**

Whatever type of interviewers you have or their level of experience, you can maintain some control of what transpires. (Even the "question shooter," while difficult to manipulate, can be directed by your responses.) Give complete answers (as a rule, never answer with a "yes" or "no") and elaborate. Do not memorize your answers or deliver something "canned." Expect the unexpected. You should try not to ramble, say "um" or "like" too much, fidget in your seat or display nervous tics. Here are some other general guidelines for making the interview go as well as possible and to make sure that you convey everything that you think is important about your candidacy:

Be authentic

This may seem simple, but interviewees who are "comfortable in their own skin" stand out versus applicants who try to say what they think everyone wants to hear. Even if your interviewer isn't specifically evaluating you on your authenticity, an applicant who speaks the truth in his own words typically exudes confidence and professionalism. Sometimes the most distinctive applicants are those who are the most natural and possess a true sense of themselves.

Make a good first impression

Even if it is subconscious, your interviewer makes a judgment about you within the first five to 10 minutes of your interview. An initial positive impression causes a "halo effect" and will affect everything you say in a good way. Similarly, an initial negative impression will cast a shadow, making it tough to redeem yourself. Making a good first impression is based not only on what you say but on your general demeanor. Are you professional, poised, energetic, positive and enthusiastic? The impression you convey in the first few minutes by your overall attitude, energy, tone of voice, expression and posture will set the stage for everything that follows. Remember never to say anything negative during an interview about other schools or people, which may give a poor impression.

Even small talk at the appropriate time can have an important effect, either positive or negative. You might find yourself speaking with a member of the faculty who is not interviewing you before the program presentation, for example. If this person has a strong impression of you, whether positive or negative, she will likely express it when your candidacy is discussed.

Create your own agenda

By agenda, I mean an outline in your mind (you don't want to display a crib sheet) of the key things about you and your experiences that you would like to discuss. This is essential because you cannot rely on your interviewer to ask about everything you would like to discuss, even all of your key experiences; you must take responsibility for bringing them up even if you wrote about them in your application. Remember that even if an interview is open file, your interviewer may not have had the time to review your materials. Also, think about how your experiences and goals are similar to those of the program and speak about them within this context. Also, if you have any future rotations or experiences planned later in the year that are related to the specialty, be sure to bring them up.

Make the interviewer's job easy

When I interviewed applicants, the most painful interviews were those that made me feel that getting information from an applicant was "like pulling teeth." In contrast, the easiest interviews were with candidates who had a lot to say that was pertinent and important. These interviewees were obviously better prepared, which impressed me because it indicated that they were taking the interview seriously enough to practice. Even though I was never a "question shooter," the applicants who gave brief answers forced me to dip into my "interview questions bank" since they said so little. Ideally, you should make your interviewer's job easy by providing her with insights and anecdotes and making segues. You don't want to ramble, but as long as you stick to the agenda you've created, it's most likely that you will address pertinent topics while making things simpler for your interviewer.

Make segues and give complete answers

Again, this comes back to the idea that you are in control. Make segues to topics you would like to discuss. For example, if you are asked why you want to pursue a certain specialty, explain not only "why" but "when" and "what." Tell the interviewer when your interest started and what you have done to explore it. If you practice doing this, your segues should become natural and conversational, and your interviewer will remain engaged in what you are saying. By making these references and elaborating, you will naturally inspire further discussion and create prompts for your interviewer.

Try your best to make your interview conversational

The more experienced interviewers will naturally try to make your interview conversational but, just like any conversation, your interview is a give and take so do your best to keep the flow going. At the same time, be sure that you keep an air of formality to your interview even if your interviewer becomes too informal. Also, try not to dwell too much on one topic or to get off topic. Unless you are interviewing with a chairperson or someone who is very experienced and you feel like you have already covered many of the basics of your experience and motivations, it is usually only an inexperienced interviewer who allows the interview to get off track. It is your job to make sure this doesn't happen.

Bring up "red flags"

Be sure to strategically bring up any possible "red flags," but don't dwell on them. Don't make excuses for any flaws in your application. Explain why they happened succinctly, and be straightforward and matter of fact. You may think that it would be ideal if the interviewer doesn't bring up a red flag in your application, such as gaps in time or a USMLE failure. In reality, it is best if you have an opportunity to address these issues during the interview because they inevitably will come up in behind-the-scenes discussions about you and, if your interviewer is not armed with an explanation, he will not be in a position to defend you. This puts you at a disadvantage.

Keep in mind that your interviewer's attention span is short

Don't speak for longer than three minutes about any one topic unless you sense that your interviewer wants to hear more. Pay attention to body language and cues; do you sense that your interviewer wants to interrupt you and ask a question? Does he look bored—should you wrap up your answer and allow your interviewer to move you to another topic? Is he making eye contact and acting engaged in what you are saying?

Interviewing the interviewer

Do not turn the interview around on your interviewer and start asking her questions about her career and motivations. This can be interpreted as disrespectful or make the interviewer "work," when your job is to make hers easy. On the other hand, if an interviewer mentions things about herself or if you share common career interests and goals, it is only natural to ask her questions and this demonstrates your curiosity and interpersonal skills. As with other aspects of the interview, what you discuss should be guided by the individual interviewer and the rapport between the two of you rather than by any firm rules.

Remember, you cannot be prepared for everything

During the first five to seven minutes of your interview you probably will feel anxious or ill at ease. This is normal and will improve as the interview proceeds. Try to anticipate how you respond when you are nervous and alter your behavior accordingly. Listen carefully to the questions your interviewer asks before you respond. But keep in mind that no matter how much you prepare for interviews, unpredictable questions or situations can arise. This is why I encourage applicants to have an understanding of what they want to convey. At the same time, the unexpected question can really throw the applicant who memorizes and over-prepares responses. To keep interviewing interesting for me, every year I prepared one unusual question that I asked all applicants. Inevitably, this question generated some entertaining responses, and I learned unusual things about applicants. I will never forget the applicant whom I asked to teach me something. She got up, saying, "I am going to teach you how to hula hoop." She proceeded to show me the exact way to move my hips. This applicant was outstanding, and her colorful response only enhanced my opinion of her since she had a sense of humor, was confident and could spontaneously think outside of the box. If you are asked a question that "throws you," however, **it is perfectly acceptable to pause and say, "Let me think about that." Most people are not comfortable with silences, but they are okay, and your interviewer will always allow you time to think.**

Make sure to close your interview and thank your interviewer

Your interviewer may provide you with an opportunity to make closing remarks, but, if he doesn't, be sure to make your own opportunity. Close your interview with something strong, sincere, and natural: "I would be honored to match at this program.

I feel this program would be a great fit for me. Thank you so much for taking the time to interview me today." Remember that your interviewer (unless a program or associate program director) does not get paid to interview you and volunteers to be on the residency admissions committee because he or she enjoys meeting applicants and understands the importance of selecting tomorrow's trainees.

CHAPTER 6: **HOW SHOULD YOU PREPARE FOR INTERVIEW DAY?**

Review all of your application materials

Anything about which you have written in your application is fair game for discussion. Be sure to review your application entries, curriculum vitae and personal statement and any update letters you have sent the program. You must be able to speak articulately about each of your experiences, what you learned from those experiences and how they led you to and confirmed your interest in your desired specialty (if applicable). I strongly discourage applicants from memorizing answers; sounding rehearsed can undermine your authenticity and thus your success. The line between practicing so you are prepared and being over-rehearsed is a fine one. Avoiding sounding "canned" can be especially challenging if you receive multiple interviews and are asked similar questions at all of them.

Be able to speak about any experiences since you submitted your application

The application process to residency is fluid, so you can continue to improve your candidacy after you submit your application. Be sure you can speak articulately about what you have done since you submitted your initial application and what you have planned for the year. I always liked to hear, for example, that an applicant who was applying to my emergency medicine program had additional rotations in emergency medicine scheduled or rotations that might enhance his learning, such as critical care or cardiology.

Think about your path

The best way to prepare for residency interviews is to really think about your path and how you got to the seat in which you are sitting on interview day. This may sound simple, but I am always surprised when candidates who have done "all of the right things" to get an interview cannot connect the dots in their own experiences. Think about the overarching themes in your background, when you decided to pursue a career in your desired specialty, what helped confirm your interest and where you see yourself in the future. By creating your agenda, you will know your exact path to the interview seat you now occupy. If you are an international medical graduate or a nontraditional student, you must also be able to provide a clear outline of your choices.

Know the program where you are interviewing

Since programs not only want to find the best applicants but also those who are the best fit for their individual program, you must know the details about each and every program where you interview. Review the program's curriculum, clinical sites where you will be doing rotations, faculty and resident interests and any recent changes they are promoting. Have an idea of what the residency is "known for." For example, does the program emphasize research or teaching? Seeking out information may be easy for some programs, but others may have poor websites. For programs that have less than stellar websites, you should seek out information from current residents or recent graduates or rely on interview day to become informed about the program. Contact graduates of your medical school who are current residents or recent graduates of programs to which you are applying. You should also research the current chair, program director or any other significant leadership or faculty so you know about their interests; this will give you an idea of the program's strengths. Read about the hospital where the program is based. Also be sure to know something about the city where the program is located and be able to express why you would be happy living there. Feel free to bring up whatever you have learned through your research when asked "Why our program?" You may be able to glean some information if the program offers a dinner or happy hour before interview day. (See Box 3: Informal gatherings before the interview.)

Box 3

INFORMAL GATHERINGS BEFORE THE INTERVIEW

Many programs have a dinner or happy hour the night before interview days. These events are generally recruitment efforts and are usually attended by current residents and applicants. You should dress in "business casual" attire for these events and can bring a "significant other" only if the program offers this option. You want to be social at these events but do not be too informal. Don't say anything that you wouldn't say directly to the program director. My residents would routinely come to my office the day after these dinners to tell me whom they did and did not like. So, even though you aren't being formally evaluated at these dinners, it's wise to try to make a good impression.

Here are some general guidelines for these "evening before" gatherings:

- Don't say anything that you wouldn't want the program director to hear.
- Don't spend time chatting with another applicant about another program.
- Order one alcoholic drink if everyone else is having a drink and you want one– but only if you are used to drinking alcohol. Do not order more than one drink.
- If you are ordering from a menu, do not order the filet mignon for $45 if everyone else is ordering a burger for $15.
- Go home after the event. Even if the residents invite you out for more social activities, kindly decline the offer and say, "I really want to get some sleep. Tomorrow's interview is really important to me."
- Take note of whether or not residents are at the dinner. Sometimes the guests primarily are faculty, but typically these functions are intended to provide informal opportunities for candidates to talk to the residents. You should be skeptical if your contact with the residents is limited. This may mean that either the residents opt out of events or were not invited. In either case, the implication may be that residents are not happy with the program.

CHAPTER 7: **BEFORE THE INTERVIEW—PRACTICAL CONCERNS**

Travel planning

If you are traveling to a different state for your interview, start making your travel arrangements as soon as you set your interview date. This way, if you must travel by air (be sure to carry on your bag), you are likely to get the best fares. Most residency programs offer interviews on a rolling basis. Before you make your plans, it also is advisable to contact programs to which you have applied in the same geographic area where you are interviewing. It is perfectly acceptable to call a program and say: "I am interviewing at a residency program close to yours on January 17th and I am trying to economize. I am really interested in your program and I was wondering if a decision has been made on my application." Though many students feel this is pushy, as long as you are respectful, this strategy actually has the advantage of communicating that you are a desirable candidate since you have other interviews, probably moving your application to "the top of the pile," and it allows you to express your interest in the program.

It is fine if your parents, significant other or a close friend drives you to the interview since this may alleviate your anxiety, but they should not go to the interview with you. Send them to lunch, perhaps, and tell them you will call them (after you have left the vicinity of the medical complex) once you are finished.

Even if the interview day is supposed to end by 2 PM, do not schedule return flights, trains or rides anytime close to this time. Interviewers may be late and your day may go longer than expected. It is best to make evening travel plans if you are leaving the area the same day as your interview.

Remember that interview season runs from November to February so you may well run into winter travel delays. Try not to bunch up interviews too closely in the event of inclement weather. If you anticipate delays based on a weather prediction, be sure to call the program to let them know about the situation. This communicates that you are reliable and plan ahead. Keep all program phone numbers easily accessible during your travels.

Sleep

Obviously, you should try to get a good night's sleep the night before your interview. But pre-interview anxiety may make this difficult. For this reason, I advise applicants to get a full eight hours of sleep for the entire week before an interview, making it less likely that one night of sleep deprivation will negatively impact your performance.

Plan to arrive to your interview at least 15 minutes early

If the program instructs you to arrive for your interview at 9 AM, be there at 8:30 AM or 8:45 AM at the latest. Make provisions for rush hour traffic, especially if you are in a city. If you are in a new place, it is also wise to take a "dry run" to the hospital so you know exactly where you are going and how to get there. Academic medical complexes are large and often difficult to navigate. Make sure you know where you are going. If you are late for any reason, be sure to call the residency coordinator (you will, of course, have the phone number on hand) and let them know.

Eat breakfast!

Even though some programs may have some pastries or bagels when you arrive, you would be wise to eat a healthy breakfast before your interview, making sure to include some protein and to avoid a high-carbohydrate meal so your blood sugar doesn't plummet while you are interviewing. It is okay to drink some coffee the morning of your interview, but if you are especially anxious consider having only a small cup or skipping the caffeine entirely.

Participate in "optional" activities

Nothing on the interview day agenda should be considered optional. It is essential to demonstrate interest in the program, so opting out of a dinner the night before the interview, for example, may communicate that you aren't serious about the program. You may also be asked if you want to attend morning report, grand rounds or resident conference; do so enthusiastically and, even if you are bored, don't doze off! While such choices do not affect your evaluation, like everything else, they send an overall message about you.

CHAPTER 8: **INTERVIEW DAY—THE NITTY GRITTIES**

The schedule

Interview days vary but follow a general pattern. The schedule generally is similar to the one below.

8:30 AM: Arrive at the interview office

9:00 AM: Presentation by program director

10:30 AM: Tour of facilities

12 noon: Lunch with residents

1:00 PM – 3:00 PM: Interviews

The presentation and tour can give you tremendous insight into a program's philosophy, structure and stability. For example, if the program director is not present on interview day and the assistant director is instead giving the introduction, you should be concerned about the program director's commitment to the program, her organizational skills and the training that you might obtain in this program. Conversely, when the department chairperson makes it a point to speak to applicants on interview day, it suggests that the departmental leadership is invested in resident education. This is essential because the chairperson typically determines how much funding is allocated to the residency, which directly impacts resident education. In addition, the chairperson's involvement in resident selection suggests that the residency and departmental leadership collaborate, an important aspect of running a department that is truly focused on education.

Do not feel you must ask questions during the orientation and tour. One or two applicants usually dominate these sessions and, unless they have an established rapport with the presenters, these individuals are not usually perceived in the best light. It is best to pay close attention and to show that you are doing so by making eye contact with the speaker. You may take notes during a program presentation but, as mentioned elsewhere in this book, do not take notes during your actual interviews.

Since many programs interview multiple candidates on any given day, a tremendous amount of planning and coordination is required to keep everyone on schedule. For this reason, interviews often run late, residency coordinators knock on interviewers' doors five minutes before interviews are scheduled to end to "keep things moving" or may even call interviewers when time is up. If a program is seriously behind schedule, however, you should wonder about its overall organization. It is not your responsibility to keep your interviewer on schedule. Allow your interviewer to decide when your interview will conclude and to keep track of time. Every program has faculty who are notorious for "going over." If you are late for an interview because the previous one was longer than expected, you can apologize and say, "I am sorry I am late. My last interview went over." You will not be held accountable for this delay.

What to wear

Consider this your first professional job interview and dress accordingly. By "looking the part," you demonstrate respect for the process, the profession and for the people who are taking time from their day to interview you. If the weather is cold or it is raining, it is fine to wear appropriate gear. You will be given a space to keep your belongings (see Box 4: What to bring). Above all, I encourage students to be comfortable; while you can't wear your sweatpants, the more comfortable you are, the more confident you will be. For example, I recently had an applicant who asked me if she should wear her long hair in a bun. When I asked her if she typically wore this hair style, she said, "I have no idea how to put my hair in a bun. A doctor suggested I do this to look more serious." I advised this student to wear her hair as she normally does so she has one less thing to worry about on interview day. If possible, bring an extra blouse/shirt or some stain remover for last minute emergencies.

Women

Residency applicants sometimes ask me if they can take purses or shoulder bags to interviews. I am always amazed when I read admissions books that suggest women should take only briefcases to interviews and must wear skirts. I think this advice is antiquated. It is fine to bring a purse, but don't carry your life's possessions with you; smaller is better. Women should wear a pant or skirt suit. The color does not matter as long as the look is professional. Some women wrongly think they must avoid color completely. As long as you are professional, color is okay and can help you stand out from the "sea of navy blue." In fact, I wore a professional red skirt with a more traditionally colored jacket to my medical school interviews. This actually felt empowering, and boosted my confidence, but these are individual choices. Avoid low cut shirts and high cut skirts! Wear conservative jewelry and makeup and comfortable closed-toe shoes (no sandals or open-toe). If you are wearing hose, bring an extra pair.

Most physicians do not wear perfume since patients may have allergies, so it is best to leave scent at home. Polished nails are fine, but the color should be neutral and your nails should be short. Many women who are married ask if they should wear a ring. You should do what makes you comfortable.

Men

Since men have fewer choices, this paragraph is short! It is best to wear a dark suit, but colorful ties are welcome! If you have long hair, consider a cut, and I suggest removing any earrings. It is important to wear comfortable shoes since you will be walking a lot. Be sure to shave before your interview, but leave the aftershave at home. Be neat, tidy and professional.

Remember....

Overall, how you carry yourself typically is more important than what you wear. The person in the high end suit who seems insecure and lacks confidence will not make as good an impression as the individual who shows up in a slightly wrinkled blouse and scuffed shoes, yet is self-assured and exudes enthusiasm and intelligence.

Box 4

WHAT TO BRING

I find that many residency clients are concerned about what they should bring to interviews.

Do not bring a large backpack to carry around with you
It is too bulky. It's fine to bring a backpack if you must, but plan to ask the admissions office if you can leave it there while you are on your tour and interviews.

It is acceptable to bring a suitcase, if necessary
You can ask where to leave your luggage during your interview. When I interviewed applicants, this situation was commonplace.

Bring a pen and folder or portfolio
You should take notes during program presentations, so be prepared. Most programs will give you folders with literature about the program. Do not take notes during your actual interview(s).

Bring any recent publications or updates for your interviewers
If you have any recent publications, feel free to bring them to hand to the residency coordinator so they can be added to your file. You can also bring extra copies for your interviewers in case they are interested.

Bring the appropriate outerwear
If you are traveling to a cold climate in the middle of the winter, be prepared. If you wear boots because it is snowing, be sure to bring shoes to which you can change. Similarly, if it is raining, wear appropriate gear. Program offices have places to store your belongings.

Bring something to read
Since you will likely have some down time, it is acceptable to bring a book. While I would stay away from romance novels and lightweight magazines, you do not need to bring a medical journal with you.

Fiction or the newspaper are fine choices and may even spark some discussion.

Have some cash for incidentals
I will never forget the applicant who asked us for money to buy a subway token. Enough said.

Bring a snack
Just in case you unexpectedly have to wait for your interviewer and you become hungry, it is wise to have handy something small and inconspicuous like a granola bar.

CHAPTER 9: **INTERVIEW ETIQUETTE**

Greeting people

Make eye contact with and introduce yourself to everyone you meet and smile naturally! Never call anyone by his or her first name; use his title and last name. If you aren't sure of the person's title, it is always safe to start off with "Dr. XX." Do not extend your hand when you meet someone; instead let him take this initiative since he is senior to you. Have your right hand free so you are prepared and shake hands firmly if presented with this opportunity. Respect the personal space of everyone you meet. Throughout your interview day, be sure to speak at a normal pace, with clear diction, in a normal tone and volume and in a formal conversational manner. Speaking too informally or using slang words anytime during the interview day puts you at risk for being perceived in the wrong way.

In the office

As you enter someone's office, allow her to suggest where you should sit. If she doesn't do this, wait for her to sit down first and then sit across from her where it seems most natural. Sit up straight and do not slouch. Place anything you are holding on the floor beside you. If you aren't sure what to do with your hands, fold them comfortably into your lap. It is okay to use gestures while you converse, but don't go overboard. Do not forget to smile and try to appear positive, energetic, enthusiastic and warm. Be sure to make eye contact with your interviewer throughout the interview, especially when she is talking. This demonstrates that you are attentive. This behavior will make your interviewer like you—a primary goal. Do not be offended if your interviewer's pager or cell phone goes off and she needs to answer a call. This is medicine and things come up.

Closing the interview

When it is obvious that your interview is over, allow your interviewer to stand up first and then you stand up and grab any belongings. Allow your interviewer to proceed to the door first and then follow him. He will probably say something like, "I enjoyed meeting you. Do you know how to get to where you need to go?" You should respond: "Thank you for your time. I would be thrilled to come here for residency and, yes, I know where I am going." Since your interviewer now feels acquainted with you personally, he may give you a mentor-like "pat" or extend his hand for a handshake. Again, pay attention and follow your interviewer's lead.

For more etiquette tips, see Box 5: Interview day tours and lunches: How to behave.

Following up after the interview

Write thank you notes or emails. They are unlikely to influence your candidacy, but it is good manners to write these notes. Make the note short and sweet and mention anything that was a highlight of your interview; also repeat that you are interested in the program and thank the interviewer for her time. Sometimes the residency coordinator will give applicants suggestions for contacting their interviewers so, if they do, be sure to follow their directions. But wait until you get home to send your thank you notes. I remember the candidate who was writing her thank you notes in the conference room during interview day. She handed them to the residency coordinator before she left. This seemed contrived and insincere.

Box 5

INTERVIEW DAY TOURS AND LUNCHES: HOW TO BEHAVE

General

Many clients ask me about how to behave on tours and lunches during interview days for residency. The bottom line is: **Always be respectful.**

Whether you are interacting with a secretary, program coordinator or the person who takes away the trash, it is essential to treat everyone well. Making a strong impression can help you if that impression is positive or hurt you if it is negative. **How you treat the support staff is crucial; it says a lot about your character, and even a hint of entitlement or rudeness can significantly hinder your success.**

Be sure to turn off your cell phone, and do not check email during your interview day. You must appear attentive and undistracted the entire day.

Tours

On tours, be front and center, pay attention and make eye contact with your tour guide to demonstrate that you are paying attention. When I was a tour guide, I could always tell who was lingering, chatting or was disinterested and who was really paying attention to what I said. While it is good to ask questions, don't dominate or interrupt the tour guide

Be kind to other applicants

Pretend you are in a fishbowl during your residency interview day. If you are friendly and personable to all, it can only help your candidacy and favorably affect the overall impression that people have of you. Don't spend your time talking about other programs and comparing notes with other applicants.

What to eat

Avoid caffeinated beverages during lunch if you are nervous. Demonstrate good table manners. Also, never chew gum, though it is okay to bring breath mints with you. Do not eat a large lunch if your interviews follow the meal as this may make you sleepy.

Resident participation

Residents typically are invited to attend interview day lunches; if no residents are there and the program does not provide another opportunity to meet current residents it is a red flag suggesting that something is wrong with the program. Usually these lunches draw residents who are happy at the program and are eager to recruit you. If a resident instead complains incessantly about the program, remember that this is only one individual's opinion and that he may tend to be negative about everything. So seek out multiple views from different residents. In small programs where residents rotate at various sites, it simply may not be possible to relieve residents of their duties to meet you, a situation the program will alert you to.

Don't...ever...

Talk negatively about another program, applicant or your medical school.

CHAPTER 10: **HOW ARE APPLICANTS RANKED?**

The written summary

Typically, interviewers fill out a written summary of your candidacy. They "grade" you on your demonstrated interest in the specialty, accomplishments, academics, research and letters of reference. They also grade you on your commitment to the specialty, personality, enthusiasm, ability to communicate, compassion and motivation (see Box 6: What factors on interview day influence rankings?). They try to determine if they believe you will do well as a resident and if you would be a good fit for the program. Interviewers may fill this form out immediately after your interview or sometime during the day when they have time. They will likely refer to their notes and your application when completing this form, but how they evaluate you will mostly be based on their overall impression of you. Typically, after you leave, your interviewer "presents" you at a meeting of all of the faculty and residents who interviewed that day.

The verbal summary

As mentioned above, usually the faculty and residents convene immediately after interviewees leave to discuss their candidacy.

It depends on the program, but some offer "grades" or scores for each applicant and others rank as they go through the season. The "snapshot" that your interviewers present typically takes no more than five minutes, and they tell the other members of the committee what they suggest should be the decision on your application. Then, all members vote on your candidacy, and the outcome of the vote usually seals the decision. So, you can see that if your interviewers advocate for you, they essentially make the decision about your fate. It does happen that two interviewers disagree about a candidate, and this is when things get interesting. It is also why it is so important to have an interviewer who will really go to bat for you and fight for your candidacy. Some admissions committees allow DNRs (do not rank votes) so if someone feels strongly that a candidate should not be considered, this decision cannot be overturned. Ultimately, the program director makes all decisions and theoretically can overturn a committee decision, but this almost never happens unless some vital piece of information is uncovered after an interview.

What is a typical "committee presentation"?

"Applicant X is a great medical student. He has a longstanding and convincing interest in our specialty. He did away rotations at XXX, and XXX as well as one at his home school. His board scores and medical school grades are excellent and his letters are phenomenal. He has a really awesome letter from Dr. Smith, who is especially tough to impress. He also has done some research in our specialty and has a clear vision of where he wants to be in the future. I think he would be a great fit here and the residents with whom I spoke really liked him, too. He is smart, motivated, clearly committed to our specialty and I would rank him in the top 10. I was really impressed with this guy."

Surprisingly, most committee presentations are pretty brief and boil down your candidacy to a nutshell. And, assuming that all interviewers agree, these committee votes and decisions can be quick!

Second looks

Sometimes programs invite a candidate for a "second look." For advice on this and other issues, see Box 7: Specific concerns.

Box 6

WHAT FACTORS ON INTERVIEW DAY INFLUENCE RANKINGS?

The December 2008 Program Director Survey by the National Residency Matching Program (NRMP) indicates that the residency interview is the most important factor when ranking applicants. In making their evaluations, interviewers pay particular attention to the following, based primarily on what the candidate demonstrates during the interview day:

Interpersonal skills
Interactions with faculty
Professional attributes
Interactions with housestaff
Feedback from current residents
Perceived commitment to specialty
Leadership qualities (the second least important factor)
Perceived interest in program (the least important factor

What Happens at "Rank Day?"

Even if programs rank applicants as the season progresses, every program has an annual "rank day" that takes place in late January/early February. The residency leadership (program director, associate and assistant program directors and residency coordinator) lead these meetings, but typically departmental leaders and the faculty and residents who interviewed might also attend. Every program has its own way of running these meetings and they can be long, depending on how many applicants are being discussed. These meetings usually start with all applicants being ranked in some way, either by the scores they were assigned when they interviewed or by the ranking that was done as the season progressed. But, despite these "rough rankings" all applicants are discussed, their pictures are flashed on a wall, their files are considered and they are ranked officially. Most applicants do not move much from the position they were assigned when they interviewed, but their rank can be adjusted slightly depending on who is advocating for or against them or if the program has any additional information about the applicant.

Box 7

SPECIFIC CONCERNS

**Does the Medical Student Performance Evaluation (MSPE)
impact when interviews will be offered?**
There is a lot of debate right now regarding the usefulness of the
MSPE. To some extent, the importance of the MSPE depends on the
specialty and the program. The more competitive specialties, such
as dermatology, still wait until the MSPE is released on November 1st
to review applications because they have the luxury of knowing that
candidates will accept all interview offers, regardless of the date
they are extended. Specialties that are less competitive, however,
do not wait for the release of the MSPE to grant interviews. Why?
Program directors know that to get the most desirable applicants
they must "lock them in" early before they plan their entire interview
season since travel planning and extended time off to interview
can be an issue.

Match participation agreement violations
Even though persuasion is a violation of the match participation
agreement, I find that many programs tread a fine line between
what is considered "legal" and what is considered a violation.
If you are asked by an interviewer where else you are interviewing, for example, answer vaguely: "I am applying to a variety of
programs across the country." Sometimes interviewers will push
for you to offer specifics. If they do, you are in a bad spot and you
should be honest. Programs also should not pressure you to tell them
where you are ranking them. Again, if asked this, be vague and
diplomatic. Some programs write "love letters" to applicants after
they interview, telling the applicant that she would be a great fit
for their program. Based on my experience, I find these letters are
often misleading and insincere and in no way guarantee a match.
I suggest that applicants reply graciously to such letters but don't
ever think a letter means that you "are in."

Second looks
The most recent program directors survey indicated that second
looks do not impact a candidate's ranking, but I still suggest that

applicants attend second looks if they are offered. Why? Suppose you meet someone on a second look who really thinks you would be a great fit and puts in a good word with the program director on your behalf. Since the residency match has become more competitive, I suggest that applicants do whatever they can to give them an edge. I think second looks are especially important for programs where you interviewed early in the season to remind them of who you are.

When should you interview?

The research on this topic also indicates that when in the season you interview doesn't matter. But, my feeling is, assuming a program doesn't offer prematches, it is easier to remember applicants who interviewed later rather than earlier in the season. When I was tired at the end of a long interview season, I always appreciated meeting someone whom I really liked, and they stood out in my mind.

Canceling Interviews

It is acceptable to cancel interviews, and large programs expect cancelations late in the season. Be sure to call the program coordinator at least two weeks before your interview to cancel and send an email to confirm the cancelation. You do not need to give a reason for canceling. No-shows and "night-before" cancelations are unacceptable. Many specialty communities are small, and you would be surprised by how much people remember!

CHAPTER 11: **ZEROING IN ON INTERNATIONAL MEDICAL GRADUATES (IMGs)**

IMGs fall into two categories: US citizen IMGs and non-US citizen IMGs. Because medical school admissions in the US are becoming more and more competitive, many students attend medical school internationally, primarily in the Caribbean. Many programs are more comfortable ranking Caribbean medical students, and I find that overall the stigma of where students went to school is declining. Students are being compared with other applicants based on their USMLE scores, experience and letters of reference more objectively.

US citizen IMGs

Undoubtedly, US students will be asked why they chose to go to school in the Caribbean. I advise students to be honest. Don't tell them you wanted to go to school in another country if this isn't true. Most students go to school in the Caribbean and abroad because they could not obtain admission to medical school in the US. Whatever the reason, be honest when asked this question. And, be sure to communicate the challenges of going to school in the Caribbean. Most interviewers, unless they went to school there, do not understand what you must overcome to succeed.

Non – US citizen IMGs

Non – US citizen IMGs must be able to convey their reason for coming to the US to pursue their medical training. They are also more likely to be asked medical questions or to discuss an interesting case because program directors want to make sure they can communicate well. If the applicant had a prior career in his home country, the interviewer also wants to make sure that he will be easy to train, won't challenge his superiors and will be respectful of the hierarchy that exists in residency. On a completely anecdotal basis, I find that many of my non – US citizen IMG clients are asked questions that violate the match participation agreement, so be prepared.

APPENDIX A

The sample interview

Create an outline for your answers to the following questions, which are certainly going to be asked at most, if not all, of your interviews:

I) **Tell me about yourself.**

This is what I call a launching pad question, which can come in other versions, such as "What brings you here today?" or "Tell me why you are here." This question presents an opportunity to paint a picture of yourself and present all of the information you hope to discuss in your interview. While you don't want to go into too much detail about any one activity or experience in your response, you do want to give your interviewer enough material so she can ask more questions about the topics you mention. Questions like this one are ice breakers and give you the opportunity to really control an interview and set the stage for what will be discussed.

Sample answer:

I am 27 years old and I am currently a student at XXX medical school. I entered medical school interested in oncology because of my experience working in oncology research before medical school but discovered emergency medicine as a first year medical student when I was a patient in the department. As I watched the attending who was caring for me, I realized that he represented the type of doctor I wanted to become. I immediately sought out opportunities to shadow him in the ED and participate in research. I have done three rotations in emergency medicine and I just love it. I was thrilled to get this interview; I have heard a lot of wonderful things about this program, all of which was confirmed by what I learned today.

What does the applicant demonstrate with this answer?

He creates a clear picture of himself, his motivations and his path, how his interest in emergency medicine evolved and what he had done to develop this interest. Since residency interviews are short, it is important to be brief in an opening question, while providing pertinent information:

1. A little background
2. When his interest in emergency medicine started
3. The research he has done in emergency medicine

4. The rotations he has done in emergency medicine
5. His specific interest in the program

2) Why do you want to pursue a career in emergency medicine?

It is important to be perceived as 100% committed to your specialty. You never want to convey doubt about the specialty to which you are applying or have someone think that you are interviewing for a certain specialty as a "backup." It is a major headache for a program director when a resident drops out of a program to pursue another specialty. Although this has happened, often for good reasons, the program director hopes to match with people who are enthusiastic about the specialty and who will complete their training. I am also always a bit surprised when the student fails to mention anything about patient care when I ask this question. Be sure to express that helping patients is the cornerstone of your motivations to pursue any specialty. I encourage most clients to answer this question both in terms of "when" and "why." This enables you to tell the interviewer why you want to pursue a career in your desired specialty. You can also use segues to bring up rotations related to your desired specialty and your future career plans, which will provide your interviewer with more material to ask about. I also advise applicants not to mention salary or lifestyle as a factor in their decision to pursue any given career, even if these considerations weigh heavily in their career choice.

Sample answer:

There are many reasons I want to pursue a career in emergency medicine. First of all, as I mentioned when we started, the emergency physician represents the type of doctor I always wanted to be. They can handle any situation and actually save lives. As important, you also provide reassurance when people come in with problems that aren't life threatening. During my rotation at University Medical Center, I appreciated all of the opportunity a career in academic medicine offers, such as research and teaching. In contrast, my rotation at Community Medical Center made me appreciate the valuable role the emergency physician plays in this setting. I can really see myself happy in both of these settings and each has unique advantages. I also love caring for acutely ill patients which is why I am doing a rotation in critical care later this year. I enjoy the procedural aspect of the field and the opportunities to collaborate with other specialists. Emergency medicine will allow me to care for a diverse patient population in diverse settings.

What does the applicant demonstrate with this answer?

1. Provides background to demonstrate the duration of his interest
2. Demonstrates insight regarding the specialty and that he understands what the practice of the specialty encompasses

3. Mentions his rotations so the interviewer can ask about these specific rotations if intrigued

4. Mentions his interest in critical care and that he has plans to do a rotation

5. Mentions that he understands the difference between academic and community practice, which again shows understanding of his options

6. Gives an idea of his future plans

7. Provides segues and prompts for the interviewer to ask more questions

8. Is positive and engaging

3) Why are you interested in our program?

Program directors are looking for the best candidates but they are also seeking students who are the best fit for their program. It is essential that you research the program where you are interviewing and have specific reasons why you want to attend. Avoid "telling them what they want to hear" and choose things that are aligned with your demonstrated interests. For example, if you are an avid researcher with five original publications, do not be offended if the program that trains mostly community physicians does not actively recruit you. You must convince the interviewer that you are genuinely interested in the program. You must also make interviewers feel that they would like having you around for the duration of your residency.

Sample answer:

I want to train here for many reasons. First of all, I have to say I have enjoyed meeting everyone here and I can see myself fitting in well with the residents and attendings. I also like the setting in which residents train because it provides diverse exposure and the opportunity to care for many different patients both in terms of culture and disease process. I am also impressed by the didactics here and am especially interested in participating in the critical care part of the department and seeking out mentors. I would also be thrilled to move to this city and experience a new part of the country.

What does the applicant demonstrate with this answer?

1. He is knowledgeable and informed about the program
2. Identifies specific reasons why he is interested in the program
3. Communicates his own interest in critical care, which likely distinguishes him from other applicants and how he envisions making a contribution to the program.
4. Discusses his interest in didactics, an important part of residency training
5. Mentions that he wants to move to the city in which the program is located

Where do you see yourself in the future?

Many program directors will ask you about your future plans. While people don't expect you to know exactly what you want to do, they want to know that you have thought about your goals and that you have an understanding of your options. Even if you aren't 100% sure of your future plans, the more focused and confident you sound, the better. Your answer does not commit you to a given path, and it is expected that your goals may change during your training. It is important to have a clear idea of what you will say in response to this question on your interview day.

Sample answer:

I have thought a lot about this, and I can really see myself in one of two settings. As I have mentioned, I have an interest in critical care and will consider a fellowship in critical care. After that, I am not sure if I will pursue a career in academics or community medicine because I enjoy both settings. I like the research I am doing now and I also enjoy teaching, so I think I would enjoy academics. But I can also envision becoming really active in a large community hospital collaborating with the ICU docs. I hope to meet faculty during residency who can help me to figure out what will be the ideal choice.

What does the applicant demonstrate with this answer?

1. Shows he has thought about his options and appears focused and serious
2. Mentions his interest in critical care
3. Demonstrates an understanding of two types of practice
4. Communicates that he will seek out mentorship during residency and thus implies he will be an active resident

APPENDIX B

Other "popular" questions

1) **Tell me about a negative aspect of our specialty.**

The interviewer may also try to get a sense of your full understanding of your specialty. By asking about the negatives, he acknowledges that the specialty is not perfect. The wrong answer is "there are no negatives." This would demonstrate lack of insight.

Sample answer:

I think that it is sometimes frustrating when, as an emergency physician, you can't help the patient fully on your own and need to call in a specialist. I think that sometimes the perception is that we can't handle everything. But, I think one of the key things about EM is that you must know when you need help.

What does the applicant demonstrate with this answer?

1) Is honest and authentic

2) Presents a positive side to what he sees as a negative. Conveys that he is not perfect and demonstrates humility

2) How would the anticipated issues in health care reform affect the practice of emergency medicine?

No one expects you to be an expert in health policy. If asked this question (and many interviewers don't even touch on this topic because it is so complex), you want to convey that you have an overall understanding of the issues and how they may affect your specialty. I suggest that applicants read about health care reform during their application year at least once a week so they feel better prepared to discuss these issues, but my impression is that few interviewees are asked in detail about health care reform.

Sample answer:

I think one of the biggest concerns is lack of access to care for the uninsured. If the health care reform bill passes, then ideally there will be fewer uninsured patients so people won't present with preventable complications. When I worked at Academic Medical Center I was struck by how many patients did not have access to care and that the population, in general, was much sicker than that at Community Medical Center where everyone had doctors. I hope this will also improve the reimbursement we receive.

What does the applicant demonstrate with this answer?

1. Discusses real issues to show he has an understanding of some problems and health care reform itself and how this might impact the future of the specialty
2. Mentions his own experience at two different institutions
3. What he discusses will likely prompt further interesting discussion

3) Do you have any questions for me?

Most students feel they must have questions to ask at the close of an interview, but unless you have an interviewer whom you sense wants you to ask a question, it is not always necessary to do so. Realize that not everyone agrees with me on this point, and some people advise applicants always to ask questions, regardless of the circumstances. But I feel this is disingenuous, and I could always tell when applicants asked questions because they thought it was the right thing to do. Not only was this a waste of time for both of us, but it sometimes diluted positive feelings I had about the interview before then.

The applicant must also pay attention to an interviewer's cues, however. For example, if an interviewer says, "So, **what** questions do you have for me?" it implies that you should have some. (If your interviewer is an "egomaniac" or a "talker," he likely will want you to ask questions.) But if she asks, "Do you have **any** questions?" coming up with something is not obligatory. A good strategy is to ask questions during your interview, assuming it has a conversational tone. This has the advantage of seeming more natural and sincere and allows you, when asked about any additional queries at the end of the interview, to answer truthfully, "You have already answered all my questions."

If you feel you must ask questions, you should try to ask questions that relate to your background and demonstrate your interest in and knowledge of the program. It is also safe to ask about how much elective time residents receive, if the program has a formal mentorship program, if residents receive guidance when it is time to apply for attending jobs, and what kind of feedback to residents receive (verbal or written) and how often. If you have a specific interest, you can ask about opportunities in that area. Don't ask questions that you could easily find out the answers to on the program's website or that were addressed during the program director's opening presentation. Never ask about salary, benefits, vacation, parental leave or sick days.

Sample answer #1:

I don't have any specific questions. I have studied every page of this program's website because I am so interested in this program. The presentation and tour today were also very thorough, so I feel that all of my questions have been answered. I also peppered the residents with questions at the dinner last night! I would be really happy to train here and think it would be a great fit for me. If I think of any additional questions after I leave, to whom should I address these? Thanks for everything.

What does the applicant demonstrate with this answer?

1. Communicates to the interviewer that he prepared for the interview
2. Communicates to the interviewer that he is informed about the program
3. Demonstrates honesty and authenticity
4. Transforms the question into a statement about his enthusiasm for the program
5. By making this transformation the interviewer forgets what he asked the applicant in the first place
6. Expresses gratitude for being considered and interviewed

Sample answer #2:

Most of my questions have been addressed today and I must say that I think this program is the perfect fit for me. But, I was wondering how many residents actually take advantage of the critical care track opportunities that are available since that is what interests me, and do any residents pursue fellowships in critical care?

What does the applicant demonstrate with this answer?

1.   Communicates that he is prepared
2.   Expresses his interest in the program
3.   Curiosity about something that is related to his interest
4.   That he plans on taking on a significant role while in training

4)   What is your greatest weakness?

Personally, I can't stand this question and never asked it. I find that it is typically the unskilled interviewer who poses this question, but residency applicants are always nervous about fielding this question. Most often, applicants are advised to choose a strength that is actually a weakness, such as "I am a perfectionist." "I have a tough time saying no to opportunities." "I sometimes work so hard that I sacrifice my free time."

I suggest simply being sincere. Give a real, honest answer but not one that would be a deal breaker for residency, such as "I can't work on teams."

Sample answer:

I tend to procrastinate. I am constantly trying to improve this weakness because my procrastination causes me a lot of stress. And, when I get stressed because I am close to a deadline or exam, I am not very pleasant to be around. But, this stress is also what motivates me to get the job done.

What does the applicant demonstrate with this answer?

1. Cites a real weakness
2. Gives it a positive "spin"
3. Appears authentic and genuine

5) A patient presents to your emergency department complaining of nausea. You check her pregnancy test and she is pregnant. Her exam is otherwise normal except you notice she has several bruises on her arms and back and she says she recently fell. Her boyfriend is in the waiting room and the nurse has told you that he wants to know what is going on. The patient tells you that she does not want the boyfriend to know that she is pregnant because she wants

an abortion and he will be opposed to this. What do you do?

Ethical and "behavioral" questions can be tough. The "right" answers are not always obvious, and the key is to consider all aspects of the described situation and to consider what is in the best interest of the patient. The interviewer is looking for your "answer," of course, but he is also interested in your thought process, reasoning, ability to verbalize and to identify the issues and be sensitive to them, and whether you communicate that you are compassionate and considerate. Typically these types of questions are also designed to evaluate your professionalism, ability to work as a member of a team and cultural competence.

Sample answer:

This is a tough question. My first concern is my patient and I would need to protect her privacy and therefore would not discuss her diagnosis, treatment or care with the boyfriend or while the boyfriend was present. I would also be concerned about domestic violence in this patient and would be sure to speak with her alone and ask her about the bruises that I have noticed. If I was concerned that the patient was a victim of abuse and she was unwilling to speak openly with me, I might call in a social worker. I would also be sure to do a pelvic exam and check for sexually transmitted diseases and educate the patient about the risks of not using birth control. I would need to make sure I wasn't accusatory towards the boyfriend, however, since it is important not to jump to conclusions. I would provide the patient with the necessary resources for an abortion and for follow prenatal care. Assuming the patient was discharged, I would need to make sure the patient had resources in the event that she changed her mind about having an abortion. I would also make sure she know how to follow up regarding her lab results.

What does the applicant demonstrate with this answer?

1. Considers this situation from multiple perspectives
2. Considers how his actions will impact not only the patient but her boyfriend
3. That he thinks clearly and objectively
4. Compassion, empathy, professionalism and an understanding of the complexities of the situation
5. That he has an open mind
6. Understands that he must provide his patients with resources and follow up care

APPENDIX C

Other topics/questions you may be asked

I do not pose answers to the following potpourri of questions or topics you may be asked to address because I strongly discourage applicants from simply telling interviewers what they think they want to hear. How you deal with the following will depend on your background and experiences; demonstrating authenticity, honesty and consistency are key, so should any of these questions/subjects come up, address them in a fashion that is consistent with your application and letters of reference.

If you had a free day what would you do?

How do you achieve balance in your life?

Tell me a joke.

Teach me something.

What experience(s) made you want to pursue this specialty?

How would your best friend describe you? What would he or she say is your greatest weakness?

Tell me about an interesting case.

What is the one thing you tried really hard at but didn't turn out as expected or what has been your greatest challenge?

Did you ever have to work to help support yourself or fund your education?

How do you remember everything you have to do?

Would you change anything in your background? What and why?

Tell me about your research/clinical work/volunteer experience.

Explain your academic path.

What strengths would you bring to our program?

Explain your poor grade/USMLE/academic performance.

Tell me about an ethical dilemma.

What qualities do you possess that will help you to become a great XXX specialist?

Tell me about the most influential person in your life.

Tell me about your most valued mentor.

What is your most significant accomplishment?

What leadership roles have you held?

Why should we choose you?

How should I describe you to other members of the admissions committee?

Describe your perfect day.

Where do you see yourself in the future (10, 20 or 30 years)?

If you could change anything about your education, what would that be and why?

What kinds of books do you read? Tell me about the book you read most recently.

What do you do for fun?

In closing, is there anything else you would like to tell me?

APPENDIX D

Questions to ask the program director and faculty

General

What are the strengths and weaknesses of the program?

How would you describe a typical resident?

What do most residents do after graduation?

Do you anticipate any future changes in the program or department during the time that I would be a resident here?

How is the camaraderie between faculty and residents?

When was the program last accredited?

Is there guidance for job/fellowship searches?

What is the department's philosophy and attitude toward education?

Evaluation

How are residents evaluated?

How often are residents evaluated?

Do you have a formal advising or mentorship program?

Curriculum

Do residents have the opportunity to do electives?

Is there a scholarly project and/or research requirement?

Teaching

Is there bedside teaching?

Do faculty actively participate in resident education?

What percentage of lectures/teaching is done by residents?

Faculty

How significant is faculty turnover?

What percentage of your faculty are women?

Residents

Do residents participate in research?

Are residents involved in national committees?

Are residents encouraged to attend national meetings?

Have any residents recently left the program?

How do residents perform on board exams?

Patients

What are the demographics of the patient population?

What are the common diseases/cases here?

APPENDIX E

Questions to ask the residents

General
How would you describe the program?

Are you happy?

Do you feel you are getting excellent training?

Where do most residents live?

How is the camaraderie between residents?

Is the program concerned not only with resident education but also with resident well being?

What are the strengths and weaknesses of the program?

Why did you choose this program?

Now that you are a resident, do you feel that the presentation and interview day fairly reflected what to expect from the program?

How would you describe the residency leadership?

Has anyone been asked to leave the residency? Why?

Teaching
How is the quality of didactics?

Is there bedside teaching?

Is most of the teaching done by attendings or your fellow residents?

Curriculum

Is the curriculum well defined?

Are conferences well organized?

Do you have outside speakers?

Does the program allow for a progressive increase in responsibility over the course of the residency?

What percentage of conference time is filled with presentations by residents versus faculty?

Clinical work

What are the strengths of the various clinical sites?

What types of patients and cases do you see?

Do you feel you are seeing a good variety of cases?

Do you think the clinical environment here will prepare you to become a great attending?

What types of procedures do you do and how many? (if applicable)

APPENDIX F

A Sample Thank You Note

Dear Dr. XXX,

I want to thank you for taking the time to interview me on January 6th. I was very impressed with the residency program at Academic Medical Center. Not only do I admire the faculty's dedication to teaching but I also appreciate that I would have the opportunity to pursue my interest in critical care through the track that is offered. I also enjoyed comparing notes on our travels to India, and I hope you have a great time on your trip to Guatemala this spring. I think I would really enjoy living in XXX and feel I would be a great fit for your program. I would be honored to train with you and hope we can work together in the future.

Sincerely,

XXX

What does this applicant do?

1. He reminds the interviewer of his interview date and says thank you.
2. He reminds the interviewer of his interest in critical care.

3. He touches on a personal aspect of the conversation he had with the interviewer.

4. He conveys that he would be a good fit for the program.

"I think what we talked about regarding interviews made a huge dif-ference- I had a very cohesive story to tell and was better prepared for the last two interviews- I wish I had known about you sooner before I had my earlier interviews! I felt as if God had sent you to us. Again, my deepest thanks". [Follow up: Applicant matriculated at their first choice school where they interviewed after prepping with Dr. Freedman.]

"Dr. Freedman has been wonderfully helpful and supportive throughout the AMCAS process. Dr. Freedman did do a lot for not only me this year, but also my family (sisters, parents and grandpar-ents) who have been watching me struggle with medical school applications these last two years. Her aim is find out what drives a pre-medical student to become a future physician, and single out qualities that make an applicant unique. I received help with editing my activities section and personal statement, as well as practiced interviewing with Dr. Freedman. Her help allowed me to express my passion for the field and to better articulate the strength of my application. More importantly, she helped me realize that I was an asset to the field. After being rejected two times from medical schools, despite a good gpa and solid mcat scores, I felt that there was something inherently wrong with me. After picking apart my application, Dr. Freedman pointed out where and why schools were overlooking my application... Mock interviews with Dr. Freedman gave me confidence to approach interviews with an attitude of eagerness to learn rather than a self-contained, reticent disposition. I will be entering an excellent medical school next year, and my gratitude to Dr. Freedman and MedEdits for their help is endless. I recommend her services to anyone who is eager to pursue medicine with a drive to help better the healthcare field, and the quality of patient care."

"Before speaking with Dr. Freedman, I was under the assumption that the application process itself did not matter and that my work and scores would speak for themselves. This was not the case and sadly I learned the hard way when I was rejected by all medical schools my first round. Then, I hired Dr. Freedman. After using Dr. Freedman's services to prepare for my first interview during my second round of applying, I realized how important it was to unveil and highlight my best qualities. The application process is critical as it is your opportunity to show who you are. Dr. Freedman convinced me of this and helped me to perfect my self-presentation. Throughout the application process, she was always available, flexible and responsive to every query. Furthermore, I always feel at ease in our conversations and absolutely trust every piece of advice she offers. She is never wrong! I ended up getting into my first choice school and am thrilled with the results of her counseling. I definitely intend to use Dr. Freedman's assistance for my residency process.Thank you again, Dr. Freedman!"

"I GOT INTO MEDICAL SCHOOL!!! Thank you so much. I cannot tell you how much it has meant to have your support, Dr. Freedman. Looking back on this process, there was no one that offered better advice or preparation for my essays and the interview. It was such a great advantage to have your insider's knowledge of the admission system and without a doubt it helped me greatly... I have already told all of my friends about Dr. Freedman. But, I can honestly say that without D. Freedman's help I do not think I would have had half the success I had. There are a millions of nuances involved with medical school admissions. Dr. Freedman has the valuable experience and she will truly dedicate herself to your application... The admission process is very long and challenging. By having Dr. Freedman on my side I had an advisor focused on my application. She provided detailed help at every stage of the process. Working with Dr. Freedman made me certain that I was doing everything I could to get into medical school. She has hundreds of tips from her years working in admissions that really make the difference."